Body Codes. How the Brain Interprets the body in Numbers

Part 1

The Critical Decision-Making Process.

David Gomadza

The First Global President of the World

www.twofuture.world

PAPERBACK ISBN: 9798874128289

Body Codes. How the Brain Interprets the body in Numbers. Part 1 The Critical Decision-Making Process.

DEDICATION

To a better tomorrow for everyone.

Body Codes. How the Brain Interprets the body in Numbers. Part 1 The Critical Decision-Making Process.

CONTENTS

ACKNOWLEDGMENTS

A big thanks to Tomorrow's World Order.

INTRODUCTION.

THE CRITICAL DECISION MAKING PROCESS. ASSIGNING AND CHOOSING NUMBERS AND FINDING THE CONTEXT.

The brain assigns numbers to everything it comes across. These things it comes into contact with are all categorized according to a certain criterion. Something the brain will use to speed up the thinking process and the reactions time. The body must anticipate what a person is going to do next and quickly set everything in place for the brain's thoughts to be executed as fast as possible.

The body controls everything that happens to a person since birth in numbers. Everything is numbered and categorized so that the brain can just pick a number related to that action or function and choose the correct category.

The brain will create a template with all these numbers and simply assigns a correct category.

The body will forever use these numbers.

Firstly, I will look at the critical decision process and how the brain assign values to likely response in search of the correct answer using the context as the guide line. The brain categorize critical thinking functions into numbers from one to twenty based on context, action and context. All critical questions, functions and actions are grouped into groups from 1 to 20. Now the brain can easy select group 8 with everything to do with the creator or someone in authority who might answer questions we don't have solutions to. If a person is thinking about the creator the brain will simply select number 8 and then try to find the context using the method below. It eliminates all the wrong responses and places the likely outcome based on a value of either 10 or -10. It then adds up things like nerve impulses to the context. This first part of the book will look at the critical decision making and the identification of the context. Part II of the book will deal with body numbers on a large scale.

A Brain Decoder

A brain decoder explains what the brain is thinking about but not in real time. If one wants to know exactly how to decode the brain in real time, then one must get a brain emulfision

Read also this book.

Brain-Digital Dicepher-Digital Analogue-Digital Impulses to Brain Action Potentials-Computer/Smartphone-Interface

Thoughts to Smartphone/Machine App
David Gomadza

https://play.google.com/store/books/details/David_Gomadza_Brai n_Digital_Dicepher_Digital_Analo?id=_rvrEAAAQBAJ&hl=en_G B&gl=US

A brain decoder is needed to determine the context of the number as a number might have a lot of actions and functions surrounding it and all meaning differently based on the context in which this is used. The brain decoder will tell us in what category the context lies.

1. how are you
    where have you been
    what have you been up to
    what have you been doing
    what kind of things you like
    have you been seen
    what can I do for you
    have you been talked to already
    ah yes
    ok
    what
    I am

not
think
what if
have you been
what have you been
ask and don't
where and how
do you normally
also
as if
what if ---then what
oh
yes
yes then what after
can i
ah I see
do you want me
ok
ok what
then
two
my name is
because
where have you
where were you been
what then if i say
oh weather
then
what is what if
then what
if I and if you
if we can yes we can
can i?
what can i?
can I and if you
where is
where was
where then
we do

what
was
when
if we
then what
do - we
do - they
do - her
do – he

2 hey
can i ask
can we ask
can they ask
can he ask
can he or she
can they ask as well
can we ask as well
can she ask as well
can he ask as well
what if he can
what if she can
what can they
what is what that they can –
what was then
what is now
what was then
what if then
what was then – if now is different
what then
is he
was he
was she
is she
was she then
is she now
was she then – if now she is
i am
if you are then what

if you - then who
what then is
what is then
what was then if now is this
what now if then it was this
if you can then we can do like
what can you say if we say
what can he do if we can
what is now
who is
who then – if
if we then how what was and what is
if you ask now what can happen then
if we can then can we
has we not been informed
can we do
how can we if we can
has he been
has she been
has they been
has they been – if
what about he
what about she
what about us
what about they
what about who
what about if we
if they - then what
if he – then what
is she - then what
today can we
yesterday did we
today did they
when do they _ if we
what can be _ if we
can we if they we can't
do they if they can't
what was then - is what now
if we all what then

can we ask all what we can – do
can we go and come back
can we go
can they go
do they go and where
where can they go
can they go alone
can they go with us
what is that you want doing
can they do that - if we
can he do that - if he
can she do that – if she
can she
can he
can they
can those
can these
can all
if we - then what
if they - then what
if he - then what
if she - then what
can we - if what
what can - if we
what can - if they
what can - if those
what can - if what
what can – if they do
what if they can
what is that
what was that
what then if
what was then
what is now
can we - if they
was she – do they
what is then – do they
where was
was there

was is there
what then if we
what was then if they
what was then if those
what was then f these
what is what
what was what
what then is
who then is
was there
is there
do they
what if they as we
what can they do if they
if then what then
if he then what
if she then what
if they then   what
what was then and what is now
what can if we can
was then is when
what is when is
what can they if
what then if
what can they if
what can they if those
what can if these
today i
yesterday i
in the future they
in the past they
yesterday they
yesterday those
yesterday do they
can they
do they
was there
do they
if they

i am
is he
is she
do they
do we
do they
do those
do these
if I can then
if they can
do they
can they
is she
was she
was he
what if we can
what if they can
what if those can
what if these can
do I have to
do they have to
do those have to
do these have to
what if they
what if those can
what if these can
do they
do those
do these
have they
have those
have these
do if we can
do if they can
do if those can
do if these can
what if they do
what if these do
what if those do

what if he do
what if she do
was she
was he
was they
was those
was these
if they do this - what can we do
if they do these - what can we do
if they do those - what can we do
do they
if they
if those
if these
was this
was those
was these
was when
if they can – then we can
if those can – then we can
if these can – then we can
do they
if they
if those
if these
if we can
if they can
if those can
if they
do they
do these
do those
do these – if they do
do these – if they can
do we have to – if they can
what do they say
what do these say
what do those say
if we ask what then

if they ask what then
do they
has they
has these
has those
has he
has she
has they – if we
what is the value of
what is the value to
what is the value of these
what is the value of those
what is the value of them
what is the value of that

3. was he
if he
if she
was she
what then
do they
if they
what she
was she
if she
then what
what can
can we
do we
do they
do he
do she
do they
was she
was it
was they
was he
was she
was them

was this
was they - if
was she - if they
was she - then what
what was - then
you can if
you can if they
you can if i
you can if he
you can if they
you can if those
you can if these
you can if they - if I can
you can if these - if I can
you can if that - if I can
you can if he - if I can
what if you can what if they can
what was if they can
what was if these can
what was if those can
do they
do these
do those
if they can
do they
has they
has these
has those
what about these
what about those
what about he
what about she
what about they
do they
do they if he
can we if he can't
wat can if they can't
who was and is
what was and is

what was if these
what was if those
what do they if
what was this if
what was these if
what was those if
what was to if
what was to
what do they
what do these
what do those
was they always this
was they always that
was they always these
was they always those
do they - if
do they - also
do they - them
do they - was
what was then
what is now
what was those
what is they
what is these
do they if they
do they if these
do they if those
what can we do
what can they do
what can these do
what can those do
what can they – if
what if they
what has they
what has these
what has those
what then - if
what then - if they
what then - if this

what then if - if these
what then if - those
can we
do we
they were
these were
those were
have they
have these
have they
have those
what is if we are
what was if we were
what is to be if we
what can be if we
what can they be if
what can these be if we
what can those be if we
what to do with
what to do with that
what to do with these
what to do with those
do we have to
what do they have
what do he has
what does she have
do we ask
does she ask
do they ask
do these ask
do those ask
what if we
what if they
what if these
what if those
do they if you have to
do these have to if we have to
do they have to if these must
do they have to if those must

what can we do if these can
what can we do if those can
what can they do is he can
what can they do is she can
what can they
what can they - if they
what was they
what was these
what was those
do they have to
do they have to - if they
do they must be if
what was if they
what can be if they
what was they - if they
do they if they
what was if they
what can be if they
what can they be if they can
what can if they can – if they
what is if they can
what is if he can
what is if she can
what is if he can
do they - if they
do they if
if they who can
if he can then who can
if they can then who can
if she can then who can
if these can then who can
if those can then who can
4 hey
hey hie
hie hey
hie
hie why
hie they
hie these

hie those
hie hie
hie what
hie whose
hie where
hi if they
hie if these
hi if those
what if they
what was they
what can be they
what was they
what is they
what can they
what do they
what if they
what was they
do they if
if they what can be
if they what can he be
if they what can she be
if they what do they
if they what do these
if they what do those
if we are to
if they are to
if he is to
if she is to
if he then what
if she then what
what can this do then
what can these do then
what can those do then
5 what is and when is
what if then what
if what then what is
do we ask
do we recall
what if your age

how can we talk about this
can we talk about this outside
can we ask about this
has he stayed at
has they stayed at
has these stayed
has those stayed
do they stay if
do these stay if
do those stay if
what can if we are to
what can we do
what can they do
what can all do
what can some do
what us can do
what can he do
what can she do
what can they do
what can these do
what can those do
6 do we need this
do they need this
do they ask why
do i ask why
do they ask why who is they
to us what is
to them what is
to these what is
to those what is
what if this is — then what
what if that is not - then what
can we ask why
can they ask why
can we ash who
can we ask how
if we can what then
if we can't then what
if they can't then what

if he can't then what
if she can't then what
what if they can't
what if he can't
what if she can't
what to do if
what to do is they
what to do if he
what to do if she
what to do if he
what to do if she
what to do if he can
what to do if they can
what to do if these can
what to do if those can
can they if
can they if he
can they if she
can they if they
can they if these
can they if those
what has been
what has been if
what was if
what was then if
what was now if
what do they if
what can be if
what can be if these are
what can be if those are
if we then - can we
if we then - can they
if we then - do they
if we can what if they
if we can what if these
if they can what if those
do to is what
to do if then what
to do is what he can

to do is what she can
to do is what these can
if we can then what
what can one do
what is one to do
if one is to do this then what
if one is to act fast then what
if we are to do this then what
what can be done
what has been done
what has they done
what do they do
what will they do
what to do if they
if they then what
if they then – what
to do is to
to do is they
to do is these
to do is those
what if they can
what if these can
what if those
what can be
what can these be
what can those be
if they can then what
if they can then who
if they can they when
if they can then when
if they can then them
if they can then these
if they can they those
if we are to
if they are to
if these are to
if those are to
what if they
what if these

what if that can
if that can then what
if these can then what
if those can then what
what to do if these can
if these can then what do we do
if those can then what to do
what is what
what is who
what is when
what is they
what is these
what is those
to wo
to whom
to when
to where
to was
to them
to these
to those
to that
to then
to what
to ask
to if
to do
to that
to them
to as
to to
to is
to then
to if then
what is them
if them then what
if these then what
what if these
to hell with these

to hell with those
to hell with you
what has been
what have been
what is been
what can be
what is been
do they ask why
do they ask when
do they ask if
do they
if they who then
if these what then
if those what then
if that what then
if us what then
if them what then
if him what then
if her what then
what if they
what if he
what if she
what if he
what if she
what if
what was
what has
what is
what then is
what then was
what then has
what then
do they
do these
do those
do he
does she
do they – if
do they as those

do they as these
do they as them
do they as these
do they as those
what if – do we
what if – do they
what if – do these
what if – do those
7. if we then what
what if
what if we
what if they
if we are to
if they are to
if they were to
if he was to
if she was to
do they if we
is they
is these
is those
8. do we ask
do we tell
do we say
do we tell who
do we ask who
do they ask who
do they tell who
do they know who
do they ask whom
do they pray to who
what if they do – then what
what if we tell all then what
can we ask why
can they ask why
can we ask why
can these ask why
can those ask why
do we know when

do they know when
do they ask who
do they ask when
when do they ask
when do these ask
when do those ask
if we are to tell then what
if we are to verify then what
what can we tell about them
what can we tell about them
what is what
what is then
what has been what
what has been who
what has been whose
what has been when
do we ask more
do they ask more
do these ask more
if we are to ask then who
if we are to say then why
if we are to check then when
what can we do
what can they do
what can they tell
if we tell then who
if we tell then whom
if we tell then why
what is what
what is who
who is who
who is you
who is they
who are they
who is when
who do they ask
who do they ask
what they ask
what he ask

what she ask
what these ask
what those ask
if we then what
if they then what
do we ask
do they ask
do these ask
do those ask
if we ask then who
what can we ask
who to ask
why even ask
what if we ask
if we ask then who
do we ask all
if we ask why and what
if we ask then why and where
if we ask then who is we
if we are to ask then who is who
if we are to ask then what can we ask
if we are to ask then who must we ask
if we are to ask what can happen
if we are to ask what shall be the answer
if they are to ask what will be the answer
if we are to ask when and how
how then do we ask
how then do they ask
if they ask who then asks
if they asks then what to say
who to ask
what to ask
who to ask and why
if why then what
if what then who then
what if we are to
what if they are to
do we ask if they are
what has been agreed on

what is to be agreed on
what can be done
what is to be done
what are they to do
what can he do
what can she do
what can they do
what can these do
what can those do
if we are to do all then what
what can be done and when
if we are to ask who do we ask
if they are to ask then who do they ask
if she is to ask who do they ask
if he is to ask then why do they ask
if they are to ask why even ask
what if they do this – then what
what if they ask and get no answer – then what
if we ask and don't get an answer who to ask further
what if we ask and get no answer then what
if we are to ask then who can we ask
if we ask what can be expected of us
what can be done if we don't get answers
if we get answers then what
what is what of everything
can we ask [who] creator
if creator has answers then what
if creator has message then what
what do we do
what do they do
what is to be done
what can be done
what has been done
what is to be done
what can be done
what is to be done
what can not be done
who can do what
what can be done by who

who has the power to decide and what
what can be decided and by who
if we are to ask who shall we ask
can we ask yahweh
if yes then where is yahweh
if we can ask then what can we ask yahweh
if we can ask whom shall we ask
can we ask yahweh about daily life
can we ask Yahweh about daily life
can we ask who is doing and what
can we have a reason to ask the creator questions
does Yahweh entertain questions about earthly like
can we ask Yahweh why we are humans and not angels
can we ask Yahweh why the earth is what it is
can Yahweh respond and how can he respond
how can we talk to humans
how can humans understand Yahweh
does Yahweh need special instruments to communicate with us
what if we can hear Yahweh then what
can we ask Yahweh what is to come
can Yahweh entertain the our questions about earthly life
does Yahweh know we exist
does Yahweh know us one by one
what if we can ask Yahweh about the past
what if we can ask Yahweh about the future
what can he do about the future
do we ask why the earth is such a mess
why has everything to do with Yahweh so complicated
is there one of us who can easily talk to Yahweh
what must we do if we want to talk to Yahweh
can Yahweh be seen by a naked eye
can Yahweh answer all our questions even if they are not to do with
death
above all how can we go to Yahweh and return alive
if we return what shall we say and why
can we not attract unwanted attention as some view this as disallowed
what if one of us can be smart to go to Yahweh alive and come back
what then do we have to ask him
would others believe him

what is to ask Yahweh that is so critical
what can Yahweh say about the wars
what can Yahweh say about the poverty
can we ask Yahweh everything we need to use here on earth
what would happen later if we then die and go to Yahweh would Yahweh not be angry with us
what can be done to prepare mankind for the future with Yahweh
can we ask why we die and he does not
can we ask and tell him what we want
is what we want in line with his plans for humanity
what if he can easily change everything and ask us to die first
what can be asked about the creator
can the creator respond in a way we want
can we tell all humans what we can do about this
will this not create even further division
what if the information was supposed to be secret what then
what is to be asked of Yahweh about poverty and death
what can Yahweh say in response
can Yahwe acknowledge our existence as humanity
can Yahweh know everyone on earth
is there a special race associated with Yahweh
is Israel Yahweh's chosen people
what will Yahweh think about wars
what will Yahweh think about us as humans
can others go to heaven and other not
what happens when a person dies
what can be done by Yahweh what humans can't copy and do
do we ask why the earth is such a mess
who is responsible for this Yahweh or humans and if humans which humans
do we ask everything we want or reserve some so as not to waste time
if we had to ask who shall we ask who shall we ask
who else can answer our questions
what if we can ask some questions and not all then what
what can be asked about Yahweh himself
can we ask questions about creation and the afterlife
can Yahweh respond to all this
can Yahweh not be surprised to be discovered?

9. what can be said about life in general
can we ask anyone about life
what can be done to life to improve it
what can be said about life
who controls life
who answers life
what life whose life
what if we ask then what
what if we ask then who
what if we ask then whose
what if we ask then when
what if we ask then which
we can ask everything but
we can ask anyone but
we can ask everyone if
we can ask all if and when
what is the correct way to ask
can we polite
can we be rude to get fast answers
can we act in such a certain way to get our response pronto
what is to be done on a daily basis
what can be done to all
what can be said by all
what can be said by some
what can be done by some
what can be done to some
what is to be done to some
what has been done to some
what is to be done and when
what can be done to some
if to some then when
if to all then what if
if we are to ask what if then what
what is to be is to be
what can be done to all
what is to be to all
can we make things works fast and why what can be said as the
answer
what can we do to alleviate the situation can

can we ask if we can do this and more
what can be done to all
what can be expected of some
can we ask why things are the way they are
what is to be said about life
can we talk about justice
can we ask why things are the way they are
what can be said about us
can we interpret life as others do
what is the difference between us and others
what if we can tell others what we think about life how do we expect
them to react
can we ask other what they view life as
what can be said about us
what is life after all
can we all tell others what our life is like
can we ask everyone what they think life is like
what is life for real
10. what can be said about everything universe
can we travel to mars
can we travel to other planets
can we ask others what they think about our life
can we ask others what we can improve in our own lives
what can we ask about others' lives
can we tell others what they must do to improve their lives
what is said is just rumours but can we add some comments
what is life without news
do we need some excitement and sorrow
do we need money and other things all the time
what has been said is what
what to be said is what
what can be said about everyone
what can be said about life
what is to be said about routines of life
can we break these for something
can we ask others to cover for us
can we ask other what we think of them
can we ask others
can we tell others what we think of them

can we do what others do
what if that benefits them only
what if this is what is needed
what do others say about this
can we ask why things happen
what has been said about us
can we comment as well
what can we do in this situation
can we ask others for help
can we tell others what we think of them
who decides what
what can be said about others
what can be said about us
what is life in all this
what can be deduced from all this
who is to answer all our questions
what can be said about life in general
what is said to all
what is said to some
what is what
what is which
what can be said of that
what can be said of this
who control what
what controls who
who is who in all this
can we ask others to verify our beliefs
can we tell others what we can
can we ask others
can others ask us
can we talk
can we preach to others
can others preach to you
can we teach others what we know and on what basis
can we tell everyone our thoughts
can we reveal what we are thinking
can we say what we are thinking
what can be said of us by others
can we ask others their opinion

can we rejoice at others expense
can we celebrate others failures
can we tell other our life story and not expect them to laugh
can we ask others and not expect them to celebrate at our failures
what can be said about others
what cab others say about us
11. what is said about us
what can we say about others what can be said about both us and others
12 can others say what we want them to say
can others say about us
what can be said about us
what is said is said but how is it said?
13. what is all this in relation to noise
can we not assume others as irritated by our own thoughts
can we not tell others about what we want
what can we say to all
what can others say to us
what is that which others want from us
what can we expect to tell others about all this
if we ask them then what
what is said is said in private and can we make this public
what can be said to others to make us aware of their existence
14. can we ask other about our preferences
can others listen to our wants
can we tell others about our lives
what can other say about our own lives
what is said about all this
what can be saved about others
what can be said about us
what is said is said in confidence
what is said is said in honor can we betray that honor in confidence
can we ask what is wrong and can we tell others what is wrong
what if we can resolve everything
what can others can say to us
what is said is said and what?
15. what is the rules of all this
can we do things the way we want them
can we ask them anything

can they ask you anything
can we do what others want
can we ask what others want
what can others say about us
what can be said about others
what can others say about us
what can be said about everything
can everything be said and to who?
16. what is the reason for all this
can we deal with other things first
can we deal with others as they deal with us
what can be done to all
what can be done to some
what can be done to everyone?
17. what is can always be
what can be is always
what has been is now
what can be said of others that we can't say to them
are we not in a similar position?
18. what is said is said
what can be done
what is done
what has been done
what can we do
what can be done
what has been done
what can they do
what can we do
what is to do
what is left to do
what is left and to be done chores
what is all this in relation to life
what can be said about life
what can be said about others
can others tell us anything
what can we do
what can be done
what has to be done
what is to do

what has been done
what is to be done first and by whom?
19. do we have to
can we do what others refuse to do
what can others say about us
what is there to do
what is there not to do
what can be said about everyone
what is to be done by us
what can be said by others that we can tolerate
what can we say that others can't tolerate
what has been said about others
20. can we tell everyone what to do
can we ask others what we know if not why
what can other think of us
what is there to think
what is there not to think
can other send us everything we want
can we send other what we want
can we ask everyone what we can do and say
what has been done already
what can be done now and in the future
can we ask everyone what we want
can we tell us what has been done
can we ask everyone what we want
can we tell all what to say
can we tell them how they want what we want
can others do what we must do
can others do what we want to do
can others do what we don't want to do
what can we tell others
can we defend others
can we say enough is enough
what then is that we can do if we can't do this?

How the brain assign the context to each of the above 20 critical
thinking points of any human brain.

We have seen that every brain can easily assign any number to a

function or action it perceive as necessary so that it wont repeat things but can make use of this number function to easily and quickly identify critical functions to execute swiftly and smoothly
Now that we have identified all the critical points we must now identify what we call as the context of the brain thoughts.
We must assign a value to each critical thinking that is every point must be weigh and as such the ones that weigh heavily will be picked up as the context of the brain thought
We can assign a number based on what has been said and why
The brain will assign a number to all possibilities and the heavy laden will be chosen from all possibilities
This is how the brain will assign these values
1. the brain will assess the context
2. the brain will attach a value to each context
3. we can then add the value and the context to have a laden value this is the value we use to attach a final value
    let us say that I say something like I want to eat chicken then there are a lot of options to choose from the first one is one that say I David want to run away because I am scared
    the second is the one that says I want what's good to eat like a chicken
    then looking at these two we can easily see that the context has something to eat
    there are other things the brain will look at
    these are the nerve impulses induced with the thought
    it will be absurd to think that I am thinking of running away and yet let my mouth salivate
    so we can tell straight away that no one will think to run with their mouth everyone wants to eat with their mouths
    if we are to take the context of the brain thought and attach to it all the nerve impulses and once that is done then we can assign a value to the context and see that if the context has anything to do with eating then the value is a 10
    if the context has a scared context then the value has a -10
    if we add all the contexts and the nerve impulse value then we must say that what we have is what is said in this context
    we can clearly see that at the end we will have a value that is greater than the value of the context
    what we can say is that we must make sure that everything

else correspondence to the value of the context that means if
we are to ask what can be done then we must ask why this is
happening
we must assign values to all possible answers
we must ask everyone what we do with all this
can we calculate the true context from a range of values or we
need specific ones
what is the context of all this can we say that we are here to
defend what is the context
can we assume that the context is evidenced by guessing?
 Now we want to tell you how we can make sure that
everything is correct it is hard to tell at first because there are
a lot of situations when everything sounds the same
so that if we are to ask what can we do then we are to get an
answer that says we must be in a position to tell outright what
is the context
now we are going to set up new rules of dealing with context
that will help us decide fast what is what
we can easily deduce that if we are to do all this then we are
to make sure that we are all in the right direction
it will be a missed opportunity to find out that when we are
nearly about to finish that we have chosen the wrong decision
what can be done is that we must tell everyone the context
that means we must have more than two decision makers
we must assign one task to one and the other to the other
that means we have every possibility covered
one looking at the context of chicken as a food and the other
looking at chicken as being scared
that means we must tell everyone what to do
we can tell all what has been going on easily
we can then assign a value to each of the context that means
if we are using one of the context as the primitive and the
other as the control
that means if one is not okay then the other is
we must make sure that what we do is in line with the what
we want
we must ask the right questions first we must determine what
we can say about the context and what we think is the likely
context

then we carryout some vital checks to make sure that we must also make sure that we are not crossing the threshold or overloading the system [brain] because doing this will make it possible to get stuck rather than fail

brains are designed to act fast and within short time but using the optimal queries rather than everything

I can tell you that all brains are created equally but some have learned how to chew the perfect mouthful whereas most biter a big junk they can't process faster and without getting stuck

I will show you the best way to deal with the context

I will show you how to deal with this context

Context is somehow similar to verifying the status because you do the same operations

This is because in context you also must check what has happened before and what is likely to happen again

That means you check what has been said before in order to understand what is going on even before you assess the context

You must check and make sure we have the correct context

That means all we have to do is get the final result and use it in line with what has been said already

We can then go on to say that if we are to ask anyone what is the likelihood of the context being the one as before

This will give us a rough idea of what the person is talking about

We can ask others nearby what they are talking about but that distracts the flow

We can then add everything to previous context and current context plus all nerve impulses to know exactly what a person is thinking about at any given time

But we must trade carefully as you know people's brains are delicate

We must assign a value to each other function as well that means we must use a lot of information to get to the true context but fast

The advantage is that we must increase the speed from the moment we start processing

The context must be found within a few seconds so the process must be out of this world fast

We must ask a lot of questions and fast

1. what is the context
2. what can the context tell us about the outcome
3. can we quickly check the context vis-a vis the nerve impulses
4. what can be said about the context
5. can the context be missed interpreted
6. is the context straight forward
7. can anyone repeat the same and find the context easily

we then go on to check the likely context and eliminate all the other contexts

we can then quickly assign a value

we then assign a value then ask again the same questions above

this then will give us the context

but I must say that this is not an easy process as you might think it is cumbersome and tedious because you will look at the context and ask what can be said about the context

can we repeat the context and get the same value

can we repeat and get the same but wrong value

what are the chances of getting things wrong

can we make sure that we can easily arrive at the outcome easily

is there a method we can use to do this

this means we must have a method devised that takes everything into account and easily assign values to make the process fast and easy

we must ask ourselves what we can do with all the information we have ask as well what can be said about all this

we might ask what can be said about all this

if we are to ask everyone about all this everyone will tell us at least a feedback we must use

we must tell everyone that we are strong together

this means you might need to use other people's resources

we must therefore make sure that everyone involved have proper access to redress and channels of help

we must tell also everyone what is happening and why this is why brains might need a lot of minutes at the beginning and at the end

we can assume as well that brains need extra care not to push way to hard as they will become fragile that means not ask to overload

make sure that the amount of work is doable and the brain can easily deal with this

I will also look at how the brain assigned the values to each reason.

now we must ask our selves 4 critical questions before the beginning
You must ask why the context is important
You must ask why this is so
You must ask why the brains think the way they do
finally you must understand age related issues that might confuse the context
we can finally say that if we are to ask a question the brain will respond in such a way that it will tell exactly the context without doubt for this is what the context will have been when the thoughts were thought of

now we can look at the method the brain use to identify the context
x = y
if y = x
then we can easily say that if x = y then y = x but in the opposite side of the results
if we are to ask what need doing then we can easily say that x and y must be equal only that x is the blue side and y is the green side but also that y is the negative of the two in that is x = y then y = -x
that means that if we are to add this then x is the same as y but only in reverse order
that means that x share the same meaning as y only that x is the answer where as y is not the answer
to test this we must assume that if x is the same as y then we must first ask our system that what if x is the answer can you then eliminate all possible outcome and leave just one
that means that we must as well check what are the likely outcomes of every result fast though just because we must check everything and all possible likely results
now we must insert all possible likely results
we must also ask things like what are the likely outcome that the answer is not the chosen one
the brain will quickly check each response using the nerve impulses received in the end the brain will pick the likely result
we must assign values to everything
we must also elevate the positions of the correct values as they are corrected for example if the context is the mouth eating the chicken

then we must increase the value from -10 to 10 and reduce the other value about the chicken running from 10 to -10
this means that we are balancing the equation so that in the end we find the correct value and context

To be continued in the next book Body Codes. Part II All and Everything in Numbers.

ABOUT DAVID GOMADZA

I am the first global president of the world.
Visit
www.twofuture.world
00447719210295
davidgomadza@hotmail.com

42